RAINBOW DIET

FOR NOVICES

Enriched Recipes, Foods, Meal Plan & Procedures For Boosting And Assisting The Immune System, Vibrant Wellness And Healthy Lifestyle

DR. MATEO GABRIEL

DISCLAIMER

The information in this book is only meant to be used for general reading. In any way, the author and publisher do not promise or represent that the information in this work is full, correct, reliable, appropriate, or available. This includes any warranties that are expressed or implied. Because of this, you should only rely on this material at your own risk.

This book is not meant to replace professional help. If you have any questions about a subject, you should always get help from a qualified expert. The author and distributor of this book are not responsible for how the information in it is used or abused.

The author's thoughts and feelings are shown in this book. They do not necessarily represent the official policy or stance of any other person, group, employer, or business.

Any third-party material that you can get to through this book is not endorsed or backed by the author or publisher.

The information in this book is correct at the time it was published, after all possible checks. However, the author and distributor are not responsible for any loss, damage, or inconvenience that may be caused by mistakes or omissions.

TABLE OF CONTENTS

CHAPTER ONE

INTRODUCTION TO RAINBOW DIET

THE RAINBOW DIET

A growing number of people are adopting the Rainbow Diet, which stresses eating a wide variety of vibrant fruits and vegetables. This nutritional approach is based on the theory that the colorful pigments found in fruits and vegetables are a sign that different health-promoting substances such as vitamins, minerals, antioxidants, and phytochemicals are present. The diet, as its name implies, encourages people to include a wide variety of colorful foods in their meals, with each color standing for a distinct health benefit.

To guarantee a wide range of nutrients, one of the main tenets of the Rainbow Diet is to diversify your plate. Varieties in hue can indicate the existence of different phytonutrients, each with its own special set of health advantages, in fruits and vegetables. Lycopene, for example, is an antioxidant found in red and pink foods like watermelon and tomatoes. Green veggies, on the other hand, are high in folate and chlorophyll, such as kale and spinach. The Rainbow Diet acknowledges the value of utilizing this diversity to promote general health and well-being.

NUTRITION'S SIGNIFICANCE FOR GENERAL HEALTH

A healthy diet is essential for preserving and improving general health. Our physical and emotional health are greatly impacted by the dietary decisions we make. The body receives the vital vitamins, minerals, proteins, fats, and carbs it needs for optimum performance from a diet that is nutrient-dense and well-balanced. Nutrition does more for the body than just sate hunger; it boosts immunity, powers cellular functions, and helps ward off disease.

The Rainbow Diet is in line with the growing comprehension of the significance of nutrition for general well-being. It pushes people to think more deeply about the quality of the meals they eat and to go beyond the ease of calorie tracking. This nutritional strategy emphasizes the value of including a diverse range of nutrients in regular meals, supporting a holistic approach to health. The Rainbow Diet promotes a colorful and wide array of foods to increase the consumption of advantageous substances that contribute to general health because it recognizes the connection between nutrition and well-being.

CHAPTER TWO

KNOWLEDGE OF THE RAINBOW DIET

THE RAINBOW DIET: WHAT IS IT?

The Rainbow Diet is a dietary strategy that promotes eating a wide range of vibrant fruits and vegetables to improve general health and well-being. Its foundation is the notion that distinct groupings of nutrients, each of which contributes to a particular aspect of health, are represented by different colors in food. This diet encourages people to incorporate foods from all color categories into their daily meals, resulting in a plate that is both visually appealing and nutrient-dense.

THE HISTORY AND DEVELOPMENT OF THE RAINBOW DIET

The Rainbow Diet has its roots in the more general idea of a plant-based diet, which medical professionals have supported due to its capacity to both prevent and treat chronic illnesses. The Rainbow Diet has changed over time to include a more concentrated emphasis on the wide variety of phytonutrients that can be found in vibrant fruits and vegetables. This shift is frequently credited to the increasing corpus of scientific studies that demonstrate the health advantages of eating a range of plant-based diets.

FOUNDATIONAL IDEAS AND THEORIES OF THE RAINBOW DIET

The fundamental ideas and precepts of the Rainbow Diet are based on the conviction that the pigments found naturally in fruits and vegetables—which give them their vivid colors—also serve as indicators of vital nutrients. It is believed that these nutrients—which include vitamins, minerals, antioxidants, and phytochemicals—work in concert to support the body's processes, strengthen the immune system, and lower the chance of developing chronic illnesses.

The Rainbow Diet promotes the idea that eating should be seen as a way to provide the body with a variety of healthy substances in addition to calories.

The notion that different colors in food correspond to particular nutrients with particular health-promoting qualities is one of the main tenets of the rainbow diet. For example, lycopene, a potent antioxidant with potential cardiovascular benefits, is linked to red and pink fruits and vegetables like tomatoes and watermelon.

Foods that are orange or yellow, like sweet potatoes and carrots, contain beta-carotene, which is a precursor to vitamin A and is beneficial for the immune system and healthy vision. Chlorophyll and a multitude of vitamins and minerals abound in green leafy vegetables like kale and spinach.

HOW VARIOUS NUTRIENTS ARE REFLECTED IN COLORS

Fruits with blue or purple hues, like blueberries and grapes, are rich in antioxidants called anthocyanins, which have been connected to enhanced cardiovascular and cognitive health. Lastly, foods that are white and brown, such as garlic and mushrooms, have chemicals like allicin that may have anti-inflammatory and immune-stimulating effects.

Aiming to increase intake of these health-promoting substances and improve overall wellness, those who follow the Rainbow Diet include a wide variety of colored foods in their diet.

CHAPTER THREE

COLORS' SIGNIFICANCE IN NUTRITION

RED FOODS AND THEIR ADVANTAGES FOR HEALTH

Because of their numerous health advantages as well as their colorful and delicious appearance, red foods are important for nutrition. Red foods such as tomatoes, berries, and peppers are well-known sources of antioxidants and other nutrients. Rich in vitamins and antioxidants, tomatoes have been associated with heart health and may help lower the chance of developing some cancers. Strawberries and raspberries are two berries that are rich in antioxidants, vitamins, and minerals that boost the immune system and enhance cognitive performance. Because they are high in vitamin C, red peppers support the development of collagen and healthy skin.

EFFECTS OF LYCOPENE

One essential ingredient in red foods is lycopene, a potent antioxidant with significant health advantages. Reduced risk of chronic diseases, such as several forms of cancer and cardiovascular disorders, has been linked to lycopene. Its ability to reduce inflammation makes it an excellent supplement to a well-balanced diet, emphasizing the need to include red foods in one's daily diet.

YELLOW AND ORANGE FOODS FOR OPTIMAL HEALTH

Now let's talk about the colorful range of meals that are orange and yellow. These colors are frequently suggestive of a high concentration of key nutrients that support general health. Citrus fruits, such as grapefruits and oranges, are well known for having a high vitamin C content, which strengthens the immune system and improves skin health. Because of their vivid orange hue, carrots and sweet potatoes are great providers of beta-carotene, which is a precursor to vitamin A. For the immune system, skin, and eyes to remain healthy, beta-carotene is essential.

GREEN FOODS: A NUTRIENT POWERHOUSE

Green foods are known to be supercharged with nutrients, and including green foods in one's diet is widely acknowledged to provide numerous health advantages. Rich in vitamins, minerals, and fiber, leafy greens like kale and spinach support healthy digestion and general well-being. As a member of the cruciferous vegetable family, broccoli is well-known for its propensity to prevent cancer as well as its wealth of vitamins and antioxidants. Avocados are nutrient-dense green fruits that are high in heart-healthy monounsaturated fats that satisfy hunger and support cardiovascular health.

CHLOROPHYLL AND PHYTOCHEMICALS

Colors are important for nutrition. The vivid range of colors in different fruits and vegetables is a result of the presence of these two vital components. In addition to helping plants perform photosynthesis, the green pigment chlorophyll offers several health advantages to people. Chlorophyll, which is abundant in vitamins, minerals, and antioxidants, strengthens the immune system, aids in the body's detoxification processes, and advances general health. Furthermore, phytochemicals—plant molecules with a variety of biological activities—are frequently linked to color and are essential in the prevention of chronic illnesses.

BLUE AND PURPLE FOODS FOR ANTIOXIDANT SUPPORT

Foods with rich blue and purple colors include powerful antioxidants that can offer a host of health advantages. Grapes, eggplant, and blueberries are a few examples of these kinds of foods. These fruits and vegetables vivid hues are a result of the anthocyanins they contain, which also have antioxidant qualities that aid in scavenging the body's free radical damage.

Eating a diet high in these purple and blue foods may lower the chance of developing chronic illnesses and improve general health.

GRAPES, EGGPLANT, AND BLUEBERRIES

Blueberries, with their small size and deep blue hue, are well-known for having a high concentration of antioxidants, such as vitamin C and anthocyanins. These substances support the fruit's neuroprotective and anti-inflammatory qualities. Resveratrol, an antioxidant linked to cardiovascular health and possible anti-aging benefits, is present in both red and purple grapes.

Anthocyanins and other phytochemicals found in eggplant, which have a rich purple skin tone, have anti-inflammatory and cardiovascular properties.

Anthocyanins and Resveratrol: Anthocyanins are water-soluble pigments that give fruits and vegetables their vivid colors. They also have anti-inflammatory and antioxidant qualities. Anthocyanins are present in blue and purple foods. Resveratrol, which can be found in some berries and grapes, has been connected to heart health and may be involved in the "French Paradox," which suggests that drinking red wine in moderation lowers the risk of heart disease

These substances demonstrate how food colors can signify particular health-promoting qualities.

WHITE AND BROWN FOODS

More Than Just Eye Candy: Although their vivid hues frequently draw attention to themselves when it comes to nutrition, white and brown foods also have a wealth of other health advantages. Despite their neutral hues, garlic, onions, and mushrooms are full of special compounds that support general health. These foods demonstrate that nutritional value goes beyond the visible spectrum of color. They are well-known for their anti-inflammatory, antibacterial, and immune-boosting qualities.

MUSHROOMS, ONIONS, AND GARLIC

Allium family member's garlic and onions contain allicin, a sulfur-containing substance with strong antibacterial and antifungal effects. These foods have been linked to immune system support and cardiovascular health. Often beige or brown, mushrooms are a good source of selenium, a trace mineral that has antioxidant qualities. Including foods like garlic, onions, and mushrooms in your diet offers a variety of phytonutrients, proving that the food's health benefits go beyond appearances.

ALLICIN AND SELENIUM

When a garlic bulb is crushed or minced, a sulfur chemical called allicin is created. This component has antibacterial qualities, which adds to the herb's well-known benefits for cardiovascular and immune system health. Mushrooms contain selenium, a trace element that is vital and functions as an antioxidant to shield cells from oxidative harm. These constituents demonstrate that the nutritional value of food is contingent upon the distinct molecules that contribute to its health-promoting attributes, in addition to its hue.

Beyond simple aesthetics, color plays a vital function in nutrition as it provides a visual clue to the wide range of nutrients found in various foods. Due to their high content of lycopene and antioxidants, red foods help prevent disease and promote heart health. Foods that are orange or yellow in color and high in beta-carotene and vitamin C boost immunity and vigor. Nutrient-dense green vegetables provide vital vitamins, minerals, and fiber for general health.

CHAPTER FOUR

APPLYING THE DIET OF RAINBOW

CONSTRUCTING A HARMONIOUS RAINBOW DIET PLATE

To provide a wide range of nutrients, a balanced Rainbow Diet plate should include a diverse assortment of colorful fruits and vegetables. The idea of the rainbow diet is to eat a variety of colored foods since each hue is associated with a certain vitamin, mineral, or antioxidant. For example, lycopene is frequently found in red and pink fruits and vegetables, whereas beta-carotene is abundant in orange and yellow ones. Vegetables with green leaves are a great source of vitamins A and K. Adding a variety of colors to your plate will help you eat healthier overall.

VARIETY AND CONTROL OF PORTION

A key component of the Rainbow Diet is portion control, which guarantees that people get a balanced intake of each food category. Portion control can help people avoid overindulging and keep a healthy weight. It's also crucial to include a range of foods in each meal. This improves the diet's nutritious content and keeps things interesting, which makes it more pleasurable. An array of vibrant fruits and vegetables combined with a balance of protein, carbs, and fats results in a meal that is well-rounded and meets general nutritional requirements.

PLANNING AND PREPARING MEALS

Achieving a successful implementation of the Rainbow Diet requires effective meal planning. This entails choosing a range of vibrant meals while keeping in mind the dietary needs for every meal. By organizing their meals ahead of time, people can make sure they consume a variety of nutrients throughout the day or week. Making healthy choices convenient also greatly depends on meal preparation. Eating in bulk or keeping pre-cut fruits and vegetables on hand makes it easier for people to follow the Rainbow Diet even with hectic schedules.

INCLUDING RAINBOW FOODS IN EVERYDAY LIVING

Rainbow Foods can be incorporated throughout daily life in ways more than just the dining room. Berries and citrus fruits are examples of vibrant fruits that make a healthy substitute for packaged food. A range of colorful additions can enhance the flavor and health benefits of smoothies and salads. Trying out various cooking techniques, including sautéing, steaming, or roasting, might help improve the color of the meal you're serving.

Furthermore, choosing meals with consideration for their provenance and quality benefits both the environment and the person's general health.

The Rainbow Diet places a strong emphasis on the value of diversity, conscious planning, and portion management in creating a healthy and balanced eating schedule. People can promote their overall health and wellness in addition to enjoying a palatable and visually appealing diet by including a variety of colorful foods in their everyday lives.

BREAKFAST IDEAS

To support general health and well-being, the Rainbow Diet emphasizes a colorful and broad selection of foods. It's important to include a range of fruits and vegetables in your breakfast. Think about beginning your day with a colorful fruit salad made up of melons, berries, and citrus fruits. These fruits offer important vitamins, minerals, and antioxidants in addition to a pop of color. Furthermore, including nutritious grains in your morning routine—like quinoa or oats—can help you maintain your energy levels throughout the day. Another wholesome choice is a vibrant smoothie made with mixed fruits, leafy greens, and a protein source like plant-based protein powder or yogurt. This guarantees a nutrient-rich start to your day in addition to satisfying your taste buds.

LUNCH AND DINNER RECIPES

The Rainbow Diet advocates for a diversified and well-balanced meal for both lunch and dinner. To guarantee a varied spectrum of nutrients, incorporate a variety of vibrant veggies into your meals. In addition to being aesthetically pleasing, a rainbow stir-fry made with a variety of bell peppers, broccoli, carrots, and other vibrant veggies also supplies a good amount of vitamins and minerals. Try experimenting with other grains to give your meals more nutritious content and diversity, such as quinoa, brown rice, or whole wheat pasta. To satisfy your protein needs, you can include lean proteins, which can come from either animal or plant sources, such as fish or poultry, or plant-based sources like beans and tofu.

Use a lot of herbs and spices to make your food taste better without using a lot of salt or harmful sauces. A simple yet delectable choice might be a salad of tomatoes, basil, and mozzarella drizzled with olive oil. For added flavor and nutritional value, try marinating proteins in a variety of vibrant herbs and spices. Adopting a Mediterranean-style diet that emphasizes almonds, olive oil, and fatty fish will help promote heart health and is consistent with the Rainbow Diet's tenets.

SNACK OPTIONS

Including a range of nutrients in your daily diet is made possible by snacking, which is a crucial component of the Rainbow Diet. Choose vibrant, fresh fruit options, such as a bowl of mixed berries or apple slices with nut butter. Along with providing a delightful crunch, vegetable sticks with hummus or yogurt dip also provide vital vitamins and minerals. Nuts and seeds, such as walnuts, chia seeds, or pumpkin seeds, give extra protein and healthy fats to meals and can also be eaten on their own as a snack. Aim for a mix of macronutrients in your snack selections to keep you full and energized in between meals.

The Rainbow Diet promotes a thoughtful and varied approach to meal preparation, guaranteeing that every meal is a vibrant and nourishing celebration of different food groups. Individuals can enhance their general health and well-being in addition to enjoying a visually pleasing and savory diet by including a diverse selection of fruits, vegetables, whole grains, lean proteins, and healthy fats.

CHAPTER FIVE

THE RAINBOW DIET AND PARTICULAR MEDICAL CONDITIONS

RAINBOW DIET AND HEART HEALTH

The Rainbow Diet, which emphasizes a wide variety of vibrant fruits and vegetables, has important heart health implications. The diet's focus on whole, nutrient-dense foods may help prevent cardiovascular illnesses. Its ability to lower blood pressure and cholesterol, two essential elements in preserving heart health, is one of its fundamental features.

LOWERING BLOOD PRESSURE AND CHOLESTEROL

One of the main strategies for lowering cholesterol is the Rainbow Diet, which includes foods like oats, citrus fruits, and apples that are high in soluble fiber. In the digestive tract, soluble fiber binds to cholesterol to block its absorption and aid in its excretion from the body. Additionally, by opposing the effects of sodium, the diet's emphasis on foods high in potassium, such as bananas and leafy greens, can help manage blood pressure.

PARTICULAR COLORS' BENEFICIAL EFFECTS ON THE HEART

Varieties in fruit and vegetable colors indicate the presence of particular phytochemicals and antioxidants, each of which has advantages for the cardiovascular system. For example, foods with red and purple hues, such as berries and grapes, contain compounds called anthocyanins, which have been associated with better heart health. Similarly, beta-carotene, which is well-known for its antioxidant qualities that improve general cardiovascular function, is found in orange and yellow foods like carrots and sweet potatoes.

THE RAINBOW DIET AND WEIGHT MANAGEMENT

The Rainbow Diet has benefits for heart health, but it also helps people control their weight well. Including a broad range of vibrant, complete meals increases satiety and aids with calorie management. Furthermore, by emphasizing nutrient-dense foods, the diet helps to minimize dietary shortages and promotes a well-rounded approach to weight management.

ENCOURAGING SANE LOSS OF WEIGHT

The Rainbow Diet's focus on plant-based alternatives and entire foods is consistent with healthy weight loss concepts. A diet rich in fruits and vegetables guarantees a lower calorie density in meals while still providing vital vitamins and minerals. This can play a key role in maintaining a tasty and high-nutrient diet while establishing the calorie deficit required for weight loss.

INCREASING METABOLISM AND GAINING MUSCLE

Although the Rainbow Diet is frequently linked to weight loss, it also has advantages for people looking to increase their metabolism and gain muscle. Lean proteins, including fish and chicken, are high in critical amino acids that are necessary for the creation of muscle.

A spectrum of vitamins and minerals found in a variety of vibrant fruits and vegetables also support general metabolic function, fostering an environment that is favorable to both muscle building and a healthy metabolism.

CHAPTER SIX

IMMUNE SYSTEM ASSISTANCE

BOOSTING IMMUNITY WITH COLORFUL FOODS

Eating a colorful and varied diet, sometimes known as "eating the rainbow," is crucial for boosting immune system performance. Rainbow foods offer a wide range of vital nutrients, including vitamins, minerals, and phytochemicals. They consist of a variety of colored fruits and vegetables. These nutrients support the immune system's effectiveness and general health. Citrus fruits like strawberries, for example, are high in vitamin C and help produce white blood cells, which are important for immunological defense. The wide range of nutrients found in vibrant foods contributes to a comprehensive immune response support system, giving the body the resources it needs to successfully fight off infections and illnesses.

ANTIOXIDANTS' FUNCTION IN IMMUNE HEALTH

Antioxidants are essential for immune system support because they counteract free radicals in the body. Unstable chemicals known as free radicals can harm cells, accelerate aging, and cause several diseases.

Overexposure to free radicals can compromise the delicate balance of oxidative processes that the immune system depends on. Foods high in antioxidants, such as vegetables, berries, and nuts, aid in reducing oxidative stress and bolstering the immune system. Compounds like flavonoids and carotenoids, together with vitamins like selenium and E, function as potent antioxidants that support a healthy immune system.

HANDLING LONG-TERM ILLNESSES

The immune system can be greatly impacted by chronic illnesses, thus managing and promoting general health requires an all-encompassing strategy. Diseases like diabetes and arthritis necessitate close consideration of lifestyle decisions, food selections, and medication compliance. The prevention of problems that may impair immune function is facilitated by the appropriate management of chronic illnesses. People with chronic illnesses must collaborate closely with healthcare providers to create individualized management plans for these ailments. Maintaining overall health requires a comprehensive strategy that takes into account the immune system's functioning as well as the chronic disease.

BLOOD SUGAR REGULATION AND DIABETES

Blood sugar control is critical to immune system function because of the complex link between diabetes and the immune system. Diabetes sufferers are more prone to infections because high blood sugar can impair immune function. For diabetics to maintain immunological function, blood sugar control by a balanced diet, frequent exercise, and medication management is essential. Consuming nutrient-dense foods can also assist to control blood sugar levels, strengthen immunity overall, and supply critical nutrients. Examples of these foods include whole grains, lean proteins, and vegetables high in fiber.

INFLAMMATION AND ARTHRITIS

Joint inflammation that is characteristic of arthritis poses special difficulties for immunological function. Although inflammation is a normal immunological response, prolonged inflammation can have negative effects. In addition to treating pain and restoring joint mobility, managing arthritis also entails reducing inflammation. Flaky fish that is high in omega-3 fatty acids, vibrant fruits and vegetables, and anti-inflammatory spices like turmeric can all help control the inflammatory response. Furthermore, reducing the excessive inflammation linked to arthritis, keeping a healthy weight, and regularly performing low-impact exercise helps the immune system and enhance overall joint health. Integrative therapies are frequently successful in controlling arthritis and promoting immunological resilience because they integrate medicinal interventions with dietary and lifestyle adjustments.

CHAPTER SEVEN

OBSTACLES AND OFTEN HELD MYTHS

DISADVANTAGES OF THE RAINBOW DIET

Starting the Rainbow Diet might be difficult for several reasons, psychologically and practically. The year-round availability of a wide variety of vibrant vegetables is one typical barrier. Geographical restrictions and seasonal changes might make it difficult for people to obtain a variety of fruits and vegetables. To combat this, it's critical to investigate neighborhood farmers' markets, participate in community-supported agriculture initiatives, and accept canned or frozen foods in times when fresh produce is in short supply. It can also be easier to maintain a varied diet by modifying recipes to call for a range of colorful items.

COST-EFFECTIVE RAINBOW CUISINE

Despite popular belief, following a Rainbow Diet does not always mean spending a lot of money on groceries. Although organic or exotic produce can be more expensive, there are plenty of affordable methods to include colorful foods in one's diet.

It's practical to buy in-season fruits and vegetables, choose frozen or canned options, and take advantage of bargains and discounts. Another way to make rainbow eating more affordable is to plan your meals and reduce food waste. People might balance their dietary objectives with budgetary constraints by concentrating on locally accessible, reasonably priced solutions.

HANDLING PREFERENCES FOR TASTES

Maintaining a Rainbow Diet requires attending to taste preferences. Because of preconceived ideas about the taste or texture of some fruits or vegetables, many individuals may be reluctant to try them. Try experimenting with different recipes, flavors, and cooking techniques to get past this obstacle.

To facilitate the adjustment, try using well-known flavors or serving your favorite dishes with vibrant components. It can be simpler to follow the Rainbow Diet in the long run if one is gradually exposed to a wide variety of flavors and approaches culinary discovery with an open mind.

DISPELLING MYTHS AND FALLACIES

Like many dietary philosophies, the Rainbow Diet is not impervious to myths and false beliefs. A prevalent misconception is the idea that maintaining a varied diet calls for an excessive commitment of time and energy. In actuality, keeping a varied and colorful diet can be easy and pleasurable with the right preparation and wise decisions. Another myth is that there are no nutritional advantages to a rainbow diet—it's just about looks. Dispelling these misconceptions and highlighting the fact that a wide variety of vitamins, minerals, and antioxidants that support general health are represented by the colors of fruits and vegetables is vital.

CARBS' PLACE IN THE RAINBOW DIET

Discussions about diets frequently focus on carbohydrates, and the Rainbow Diet is no different. It is crucial to comprehend the function of carbs in this situation. Whole, unprocessed carbohydrates like those found in fruits, vegetables, and whole grains are an important source of energy, fiber, and other necessary elements. In contrast to the popular belief that carbohydrates should be avoided, the Rainbow Diet promotes a sustainable and well-balanced diet by including these healthy sources.

People can take advantage of the nutritional advantages of choosing colorful carbs while also eliminating misconceptions about this macronutrient.

COMPREHENDING PROTEINS AND FATS

The Rainbow Diet stresses a holistic approach to eating, emphasizing the value of proteins and good fats. Lean meats and other plant-based protein sources, such as legumes and nuts, should be included to provide a well-rounded intake of necessary amino acids.

In a similar vein, including vibrant sources of good fats like nuts and avocados enhances general health. The Rainbow

Diet dispels myths regarding fats' intrinsic harmfulness and promotes their moderation in nutrient-dense foods, resulting in a balanced and sustainable dietary pattern that promotes long-term health and vitality.

CHAPTER EIGHT

INTEGRATING A LONG-TERM SUSTAINABLE LIFESTYLE

CHOOSING TO LIVE A RAINBOW DIET LIFESTYLE

The Rainbow Diet, which is defined by a wide variety of vibrant fruits and vegetables, transcends fads and becomes a sustainable way of life. Adopting the Rainbow Diet promotes a well-rounded approach to nutrition by combining a range of nutrients from various food sources. People who follow this dietary pattern assist with environmental well-being in addition to their long-term health by engaging in sustainable practices.

People who adopt the Rainbow Diet as a way of life not only put more emphasis on their health but also take an active role in the larger movement of mindful and sustainable eating.

GRADUAL CHANGE AND THE DEVELOPMENT OF HABITS

The capacity to make modest changes and establish enduring habits is frequently the key to long-term sustainability. Steep and abrupt changes in lifestyle might be difficult to sustain over time. By taking a step-by-step approach, people can become used to new routines without feeling overwhelmed. The secret is to create long-lasting habits, whether that means increasing the amount of plant-based foods in your daily meals or progressively cutting back on processed foods. This gradual shift prolongs the benefits of lifestyle modifications and makes it easier to incorporate healthy behaviors.

MAINTAINING COHERENCE ACROSS VARIOUS STAGES OF LIFE

Sustainable living is based on consistency, and upholding a healthy lifestyle should be flexible enough to accommodate different stages of life. Life is dynamic, with distinct opportunities and challenges presented at various phases. Finding strategies to maintain consistency in health-promoting behaviors is essential, whether one is juggling a demanding job, starting a family, or approaching retirement. This could entail changing habits, reevaluating goals, and realizing that there are different paths to long-term sustainability at different points in life. People can modify their healthy lifestyle to fit the ever-changing demands of various life stages by adopting a flexible attitude.

INCLUDING PHYSICAL ACTIVITY AND EXERCISE TOGETHER

Beyond food, sustainability includes regular exercise and physical activity. Including physical activity in daily life improves mental and physical health in addition to physical health. Incorporating exercise into everyday routines, whether through organized exercises, leisure pursuits, or just adding more movement, encourages a comprehensive strategy for long-term sustainability. Acknowledging physical activity as an essential element of a well-rounded existence encourages behaviors that are more likely to stick over time.

HARMONY BETWEEN EXERCISE AND DIET

The combination of activity and nutrition creates a potent coalition for long-term sustainability. A well-balanced diet fosters a positive link between nutrition and exercise, enhancing the advantages of consistent exercise. A healthy diet gives you the energy and nutrients you need to perform at your best during exercise, and fitness improves your body's capacity to absorb and use nutrients. Recognizing and appreciating the relationship between fitness and diet leads to a more thorough and long-lasting approach to long-term well-being.

CUSTOMIZING EXERCISES TO MEET PERSONAL NEEDS

Incorporating exercise into a sustainable lifestyle requires an awareness of and respect for individual diversity. Exercise programs should be customized to each person's needs by taking into account their preferences, physical capabilities, and any potential restrictions. The focus is on designing a fitness plan that is both pleasant and sustainable, whether that means selecting an exercise that fits with one's interests or tailoring a program to account for particular health issues. This customized approach increases the possibility that an individual will continue to make a lifetime commitment to regular physical activity by fostering a sense of ownership over their well-being.

CHAPTER NINE
MEAL PLANS AND RECIPES
RECIPES FOR BREAKFAST

Breakfast is the ideal opportunity to start your day with a vibrant and nutrient-rich start to your day. The Rainbow Smoothie Bowl is a colorful and nutrient-dense dish that is one choice. This smoothie bowl, which is made by blending a variety of vibrant fruits including kiwi, mango, and berries, is not only aesthetically pleasing but also a good source of vitamins and antioxidants.

Oatmeal with Colorful Toppings is another filling breakfast choice. A dash of chia seeds and some colorful toppings like sliced strawberries and blueberries turn this traditional dish into a colorful canvas. In addition to being visually pleasing, this breakfast option is high in fiber, which will keep you full and focused all morning.

RECIPES FOR LUNCH AND DINNER

The Grilled Rainbow Vegetable Skewers are a visually appealing and flavorful option for lunch or dinner. These skewers, which feature bell peppers, cherry tomatoes, and zucchini among other vegetables, not only display a rainbow of hues but also supply a good amount of vitamins and minerals. The tastes are enhanced by grilling, making it a filling dinner suitable for any occasion.

Quinoa Salad with a Spectrum of Ingredients is another vibrant and wholesome choice. Quinoa is combined with a variety of vibrant veggies, herbs, and a mild vinaigrette in this adaptable recipe. This salad, which includes cucumbers, cherry tomatoes, and yellow and red bell peppers, is not only visually stunning but also a healthy, well-balanced supper.

SNACK CONCEPTS

Adding a pop of color to snacks can enhance the experience. The Cinnamon Chips with Rainbow Fruit Salsa is a tasty and nutritious snack option. The salsa, which combines sliced strawberries, pineapple, and kiwi, is a delightful and refreshing snack. When combined with handmade cinnamon chips, it adds a delightful crunch and makes for a visually appealing and delectable snack.

Another snack option is guacamole with colorful veggies, which blends the colorful tones of bell peppers, cherry tomatoes, and red onions with the creamy texture of avocado. This dip offers a variety of flavors in addition to providing necessary nutrients. Serve it with vibrant vegetable sticks for a visually appealing and nutrient-dense snack that tastes great.

GRILLED RAINBOW VEGETABLE SKEWERS

This colorful and wholesome take on a classic barbecue dish is sure to please. The variety of vibrant veggies that are expertly grilled and put onto skewers is the secret to this visually appealing dish. In addition to creating an eye-catching arrangement, the mixture of bell peppers, cherry tomatoes, red onions, zucchini, and mushrooms offers a variety of tastes and nutrients. These skewers lend a lovely Smokey and charred flavor to the naturally sweet vegetables, and they grill beautifully for a delightful outdoor gathering or barbecue.

QUINOA SALAD WITH A SPECTRUM OF INGREDIENTS

This dish, which highlights the various flavors and textures present in a range of ingredients, is wholesome and adjustable. The base is made of nutrient-dense quinoa, which provides a delightful chewiness and a full protein source. Incorporating colorful vegetables like diced cucumbers, vibrant bell peppers, cherry tomatoes, and shredded carrots not only enhances the visual appeal but also provides a variety of vitamins and minerals. Consider adding fresh herbs, such as cilantro or parsley, and tossing everything with zesty vinaigrette to further elevate the salad. This salad gives you a boost of nutrients and energy and can be eaten as a stand-alone meal or as a cool side dish.

RAINBOW FRUIT SALSA WITH CINNAMON CHIPS

This tasty and healthful take on traditional salsa is served with crunchy cinnamon chips. Strawberries, kiwis, pineapple, mango, and other fresh, diced fruits are among the colorful and sweet ingredients of this salsa. In addition to producing an eye-catching spectrum, the color combination highlights the wide range of vitamins and antioxidants that are found in the fruits. Serve homemade cinnamon chips with the salsa to balance its fruity goodness. The delightful crunch and subtle warmth from these crispy, baked chips create a pleasing harmony of flavors. This refreshing salsa is perfect as a snack, a light dessert, or a colorful addition to brunch.

GUACAMOLE WITH COLORFUL VEGGIES

Guacamole with Colorful Veggies is a classic and versatile dip that gets a vibrant twist by incorporating a spectrum of colorful vegetables. The creamy and rich avocado base is complemented by diced tomatoes, red onions, bell peppers, and cilantro, creating a visually appealing mix that is as pleasing to the eyes as it is to the taste buds. The addition of lime juice adds a refreshing zing, while the colorful veggies contribute a variety of textures and flavors. This guacamole can be served with tortilla chips, as a topping for tacos or grilled meats, or even as a spread for sandwiches. It's a versatile and nutritious dip that brings a burst of freshness to any occasion.

9 798869 788030